AF882400

Physeo

We would like to extend a special thanks to the following contributing authors who have spent countless hours and support to make Physeo possible.

Ajay Davidson, MD

Alexandra Galel, MD

Anne-Sophie van Wingerden, Medical Student
Columbia Vagelos College of Physicians and Surgeons

Anissa Laine Bayabos Amilhamja

Antonio Acevedo

Ayan Agarwal, MBBS Student
Vardhman Mahavir Medical College and Safdarjung Hospital, New Delhi, India

Brianna Cocuzzo, MsC

Camelita Thrift

Christopher A. Price, MS

Dr. Jabran Wasti, House Officer
Dr. Ruth K.M. Pfau Civil Hospital, Karachi, Pakistan

Dr. James Nunn

Genevieve Saliuk, MD Candidate 2024
UTMB School of Medicine

George Myo Win, BS
University of Missouri-Columbia School of Medicine

Ghadeer Magdy Elshafey, M.D.

H. Robert Cannon, DO

Idiel

Jennifer M. Locke, BA, MD Candidate

Justin Wong, DO

Kurestin Miller, BA, MD Candidate

Lauren S. Faber, MD

Lauren Schwartz

Lee Azolai

Leslie Jewett, MD

Logan B. Carlyle, OMS-II

Marisol Cárdenas Calderón, MD

Mark Parry, MD, Resident Physician
Department of Obstetrics and Gynecology, OhioHealth Riverside Methodist, Columbus, Ohio

Mason T. Bennet

Mateo Betancourt Escobar
Universidad Autónoma de San Luis Potosí, Mexico

Mohamed Elshennawy, MD

Natalia Kerr, MD

Nijat Aliyev, MD

Nikoloz Karazanashvili

Nirupamaa Sivanushanthan, Medical Student

Ostapenko Karolina

Dr. Rahil Patel, Medical Officer
Sharda Hospital, New Delhi, India

Mr. Rishabh Goyal

Roaa Zayat, MD

Rojin Arefi, MD

Ryan Zia

Salikh Murtaliev, MD

Sarah Jaber, DO, Internal Medicine Physician

Shawna-Kay Young, MD Student

Sergio R. Ortiz, MD, MPH

Shelia Chandrahas

Soomal Zukhruf Memon

Sumit Raut

Telyn Peterson, OMS-III
Rocky Vista University - Sourthern Utah\

Syed Ali Haider

Syed Awais Ahmed, MD

Tamari Papidze

Trey Edwards, D.O.

Warda Hameed, MD

Yasmeen Abdulrahman, MD

Yomna Dean, MS-4

Zurabi Zaalishvili

Zuka Zaalishvili

TABLE OF CONTENTS

DIFFERENTIAL DIAGNOSIS

Differential Diagnosis | Section 1 - Headache Differential

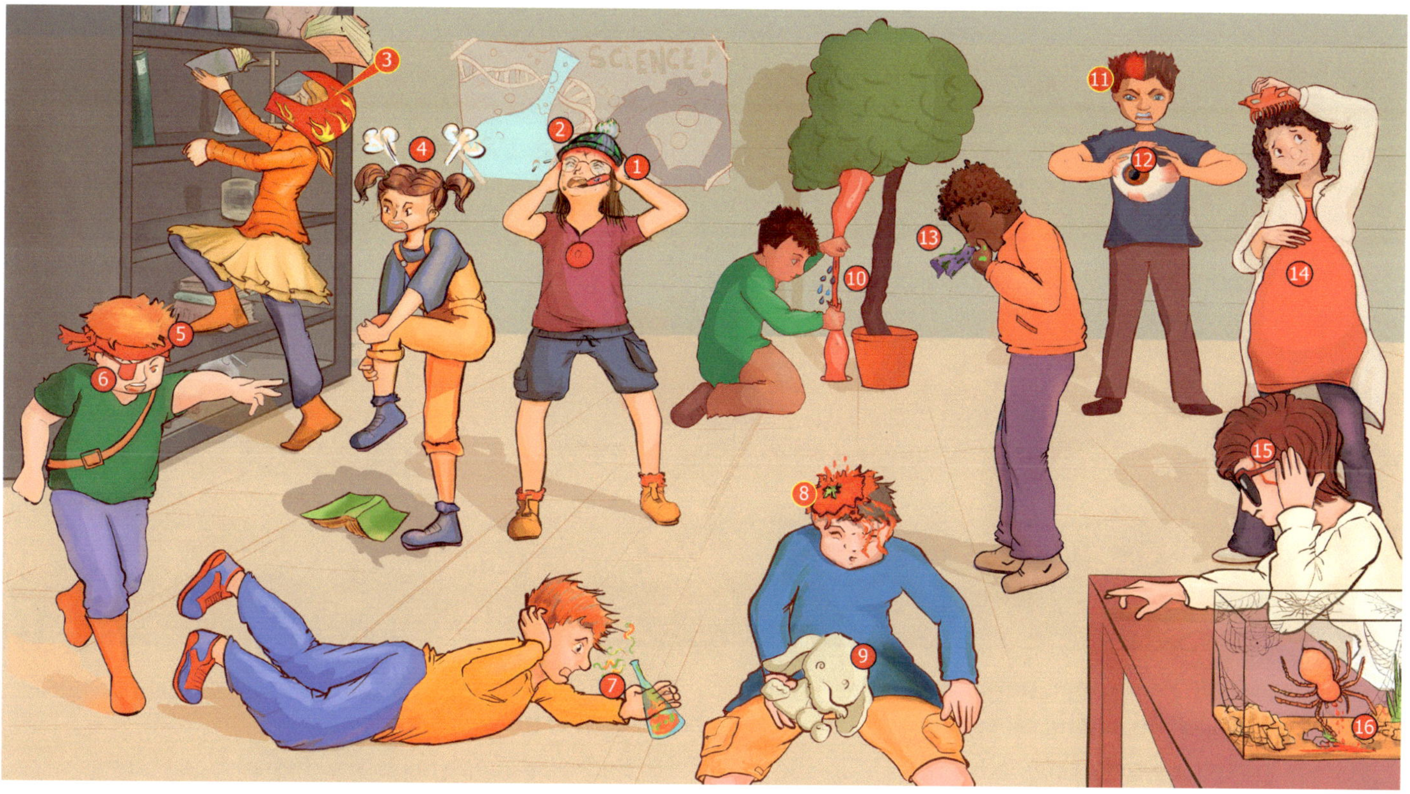

1. Student clutching head: Headache differential diagnosis

2. Beanie with green spots: Meningitis

3. Red helmet with flames: Encephalitis

4. Angry girl releasing steam from ears: Elevated intracranial pressure

5. Red bandana: Tension headache

6. Red eye patch: Cluster headache

7. Student inhaling toxic fumes while clutching the back of his head: Carbon monoxide poisoning

8. Tomato hitting head dripping down juice: Traumatic intracranial hemorrhage

9. Dumbo stuffed elephant: Hypertensive encephalopathy

10. Student tearing a red hose supplying brain-shaped tree: Carotid artery dissection

11. Halfway dyed red hair: Migraine headache

12. Applying pressure to eyeball: Acute angle-closure glaucoma

13. Green discharge from the nose: Sinusitis

14. Pregnant woman with a hair clamp: Preeclampsia

15. Artery bulging out on the side of the face: Giant cell/temporal arteritis

16. Blood underneath an arachnoid: Subarachnoid hemorrhage

Differential Diagnosis | Section 2 - Vertigo/Lightheadedness Differential

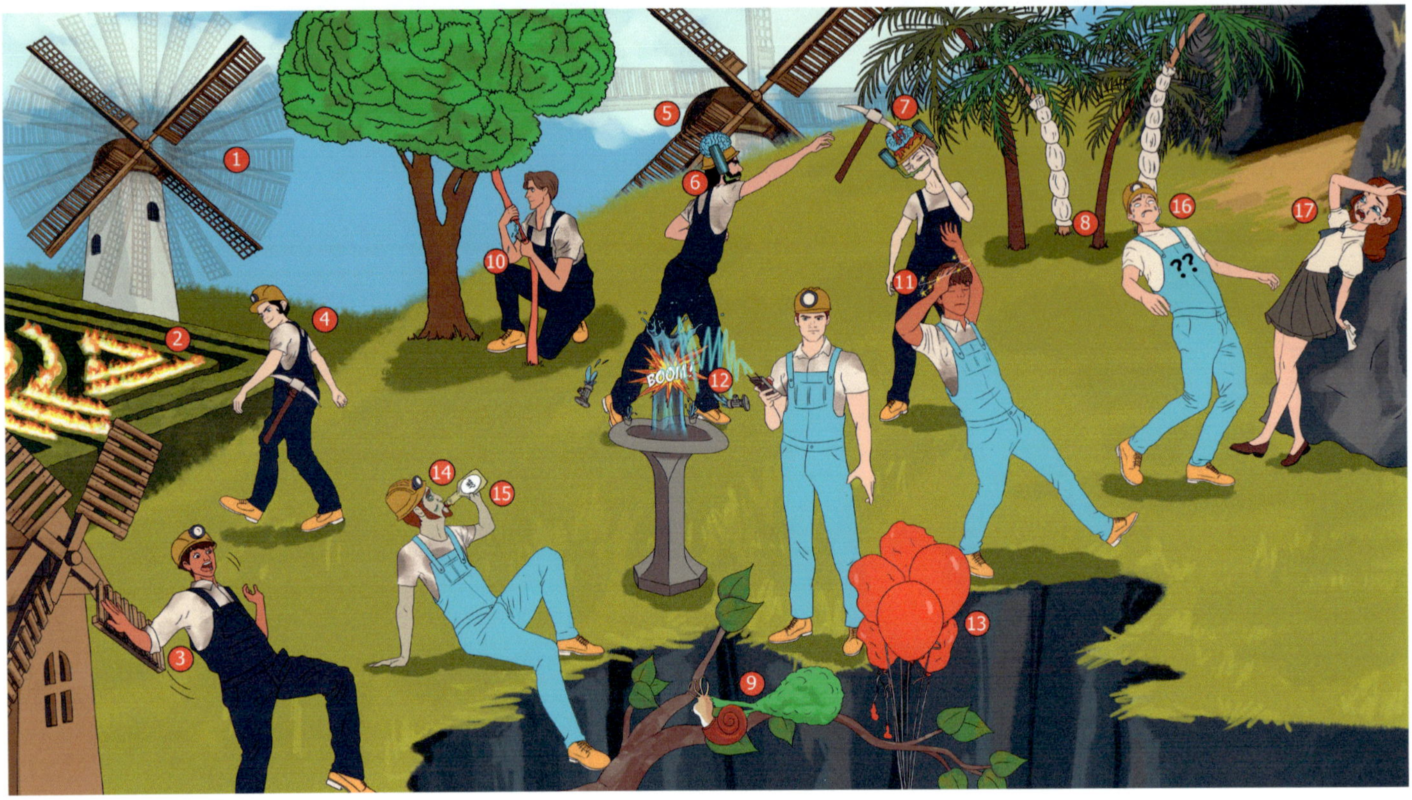

1. Stable windmill core with fast rotating blades in the periphery: Vertigo (Peripheral causes)

2. Flames in the labyrinth: Labyrinthitis

3. Man slipped while leaning against the blades of model windmill: Benign paroxysmal positional vertigo (BPPV)

4. Miner: Ménière's disease

5. Slow spinning windmill in the center: Vertigo (Central causes)

6. Clogged straw in a brain-shaped drinking hat: Ischemic stroke

7. Pierced open hard hat leaking red soda over his head and face: Intracranial hemorrhage

8. Unwrapped palm trees: Multiple sclerosis

9. Snail with vestibule looking antennas stuck at moss: Acoustic neuroma

10. Red hose supplying brain-shaped tree getting dissected: Carotid artery dissection

11. A worker stumbling around a cliff: Lightheadedness (Serious causes)

12. Irregular electrical impulses blowing up the valves of heart-shaped fountain: Cardiac causes like arrhythmia & valvular issues

13. Red, deflated balloons: Anemia

14. Sick man who looks like a zombie: Infection

15. Empty syrup bottle: Hypoglycemia

16. Man swaying on his feet, sweating profusely, with his eyes rolling back: Nonspecific (Vasovagal)

17. Girl crying excessively, while falling back: Orthostatic hypotension

Differential Diagnosis | Section 3 - Eye Complaints Differential

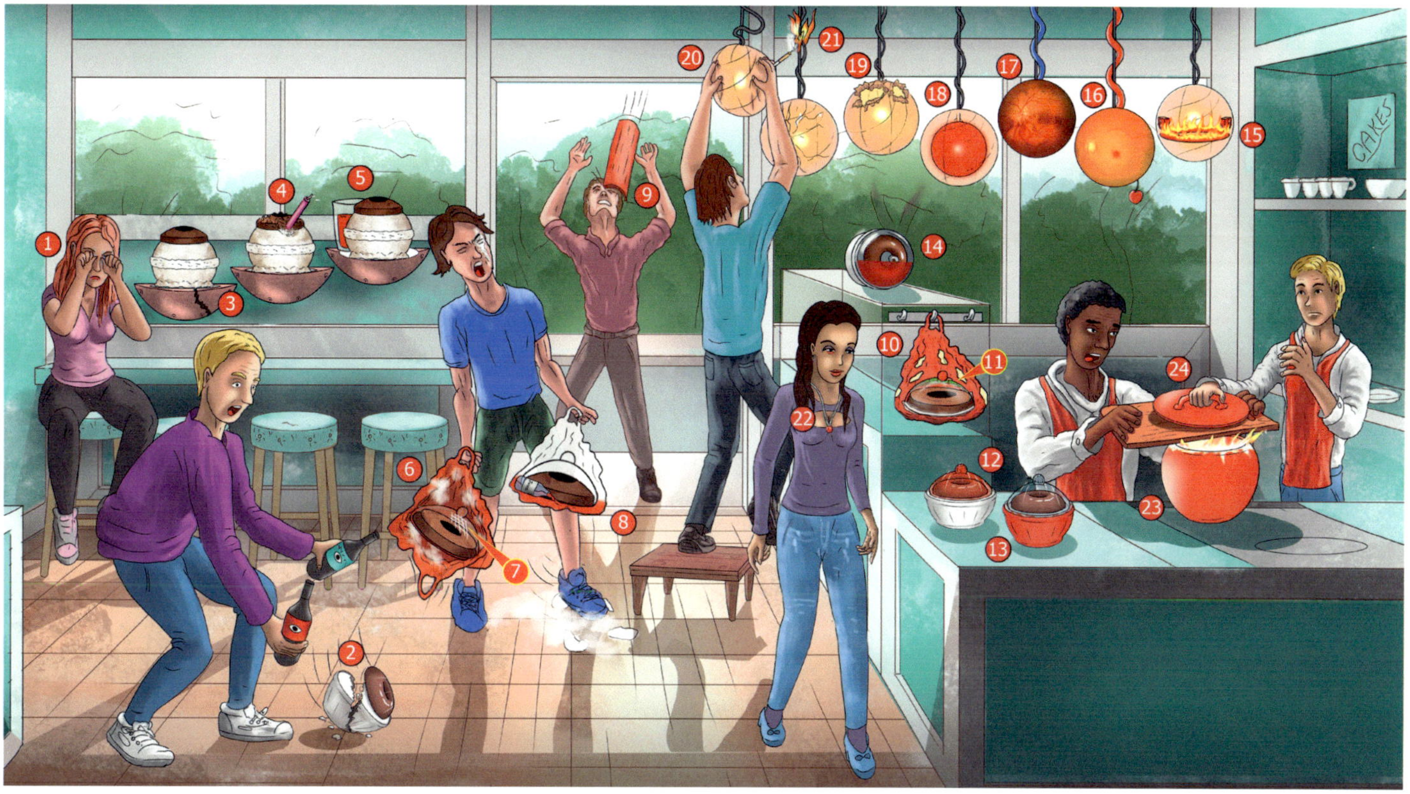

1. Customer rubbing eyes: Eye complaints

2. Broken, blown-out ceramic dish: Blowout fractures

3. Crack in eyelid-shaped shelf: Eyelid laceration

4. Candle placed forcibly into eyeball cake: Globe rupture

5. Red glass of juice behind the eye cake pushing it forward: Retrobulbar hematoma

6. Flour on eye and transparent bag with flour: Chemical conjunctivitis

7. Scratched dome glass covering cake: Corneal abrasion

8. Red icing spilling in transparent bag: Subconjunctival hemorrhage

9. Shingle falling into customers eye: Herpes zoster ophthalmicus

10. Icing rotting on red transparent bag: Non-traumatic conjunctivitis

11. Green icing on dome glass cover: Corneal ulcer

12. Red transparent dome covering white container with donut: Keratitis

13. Transparent dome covering red container with donut: Episcleritis/Scleritis

14. Red raspberry jelly located between the donut and the covering: Hyphema

15. Lantern with flaming red ring and switch: Anterior uveitis

16. Red cord around a pale lantern and a cherry hanging below: Central retinal artery occlusion (CRAO)

17. Thick blue wire and hemorrhagic lantern: Central retinal artery occlusion (CRAO)

18. Lantern with red interior: Endophthalmitis

19. Lantern cover peeling off: Retinal detachment

20. Employee pressing on sides of lantern to take it down: Glaucoma

21. Cigarette burning cord of lantern: Optic neuritis

22. Pimple on eyelid and red necklace on shirt opening: Hordeolum (Stye)

23. Flaming in a big, red cooking pot: Orbital cellulitis

24. Red lid over cutting board on red pot: Preseptal cellulitis (periorbital)

Differential Diagnosis | Section 4 - Altered Mental Status

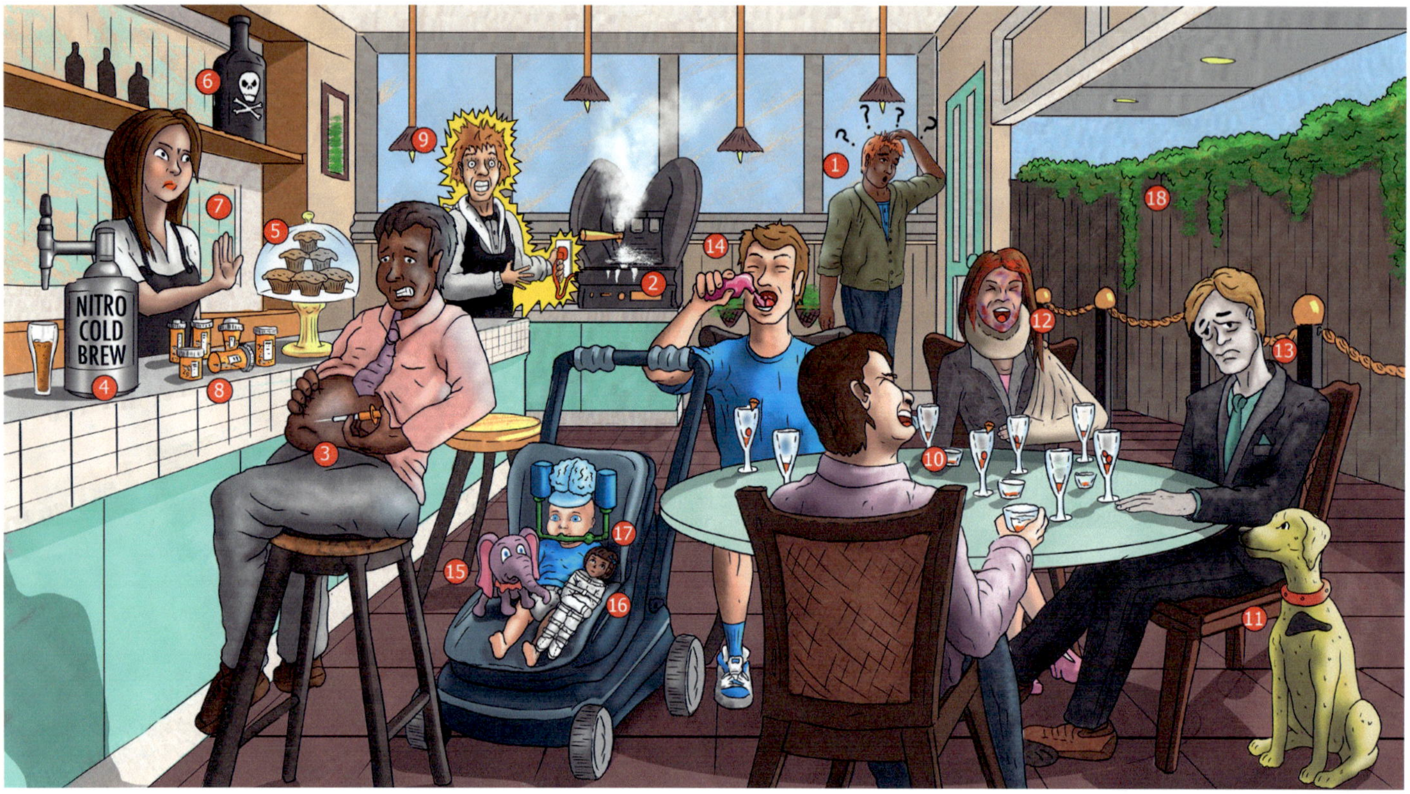

1. Confused man: Altered mental status differential

2. Steaming thyroid-shaped espresso machine: Thyrotoxicosis

3. Insulin syringe: Hypoglycemia (e.g. insulin caused hypoglycemia)

4. Nitro cold brew coffee: Uremia

5. A bunch of poppy seed muffins: Opiate toxicity

6. Black bottle with skull and crossbones design: Toxins

7. Waitress cutting off the customer from alcohol: Alcohol withdrawal

8. Multiple medications: Polypharmacy

9. Electrocution caused body shaking: Seizures

10. Empty mimosa glasses: Alcohol toxicity

11. Yellow dog with a liver shaped spot: Liver disease

12. Customer with head injuries and bruises: Brain trauma

13. Sick zombie-like customer: Infections/Sepsis

14. Drinking a concentrated pack of electrolytes: Electrolyte disturbance

15. Stuffed elephant toy with a big head: Hypertensive encephalopathy

16. Doll with straight jacket: Psychiatric illness

17. Brain-shaped soda hat with a clogged straw: Stroke

18. Moss: Space occupying lesions (e.g. tumors)

Differential Diagnosis | Section 5 - Sore Throat Differential

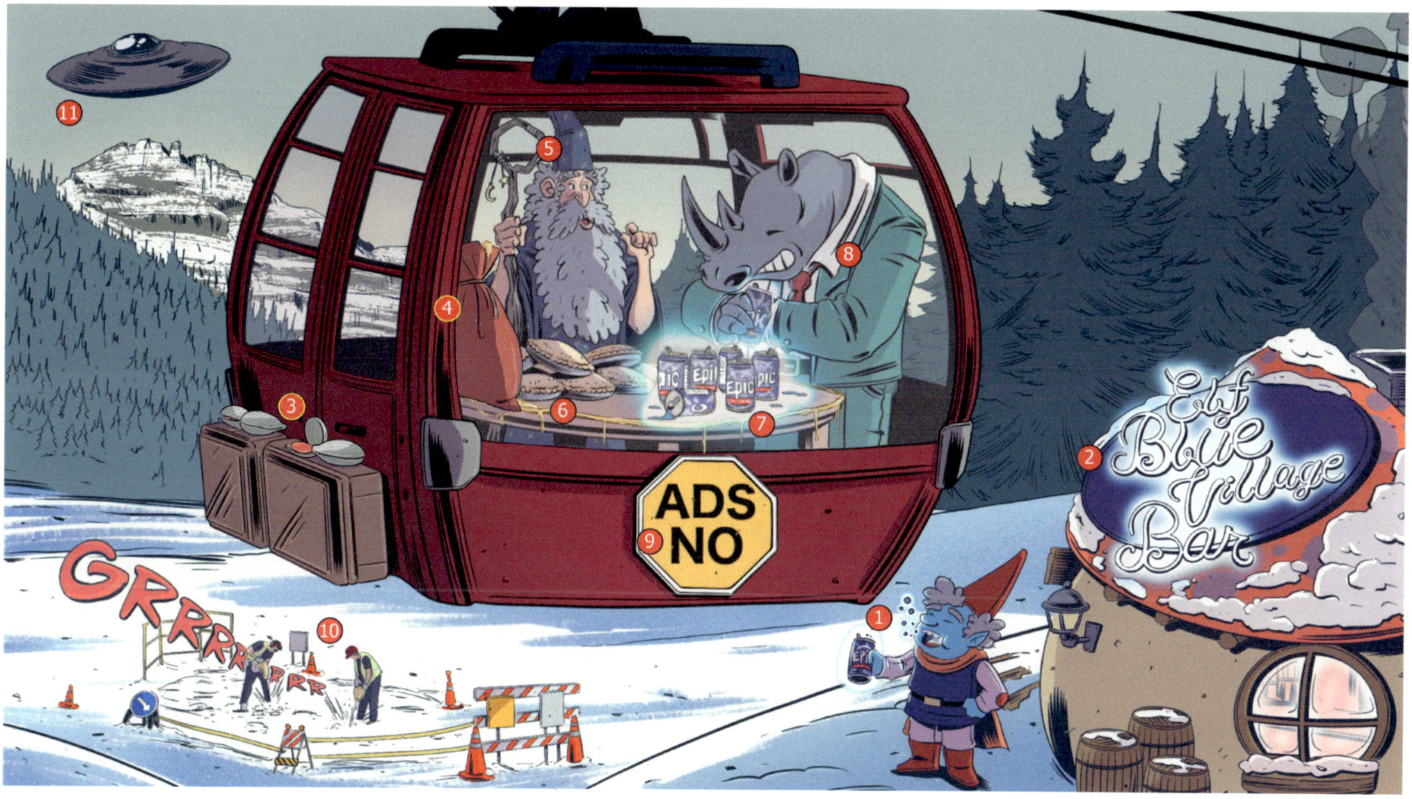

1. Elf gargling soda: Sore throat

2. Elf Blue Village Bar: Epstein-Barr virus

3. Gondola with clams on back: Neisseria gonorrhoeae/ Chlamydia

4. Sack that looks like the palatine tonsil: Peritonsillar abscess

5. Merlin's magical staff: Staphylococcus aureus

6. Pie: Strep pyogene

7. Glowing EPIC soda cans: Epiglottitis

8. Rhinoceros: Rhinovirus

9. "ADs NO" sign: Adenovirus

10. Loud digging: Ludwig's Angina

11. Unidentified flying object: Foreign body

Differential Diagnosis | Section 6 - Cough Differential

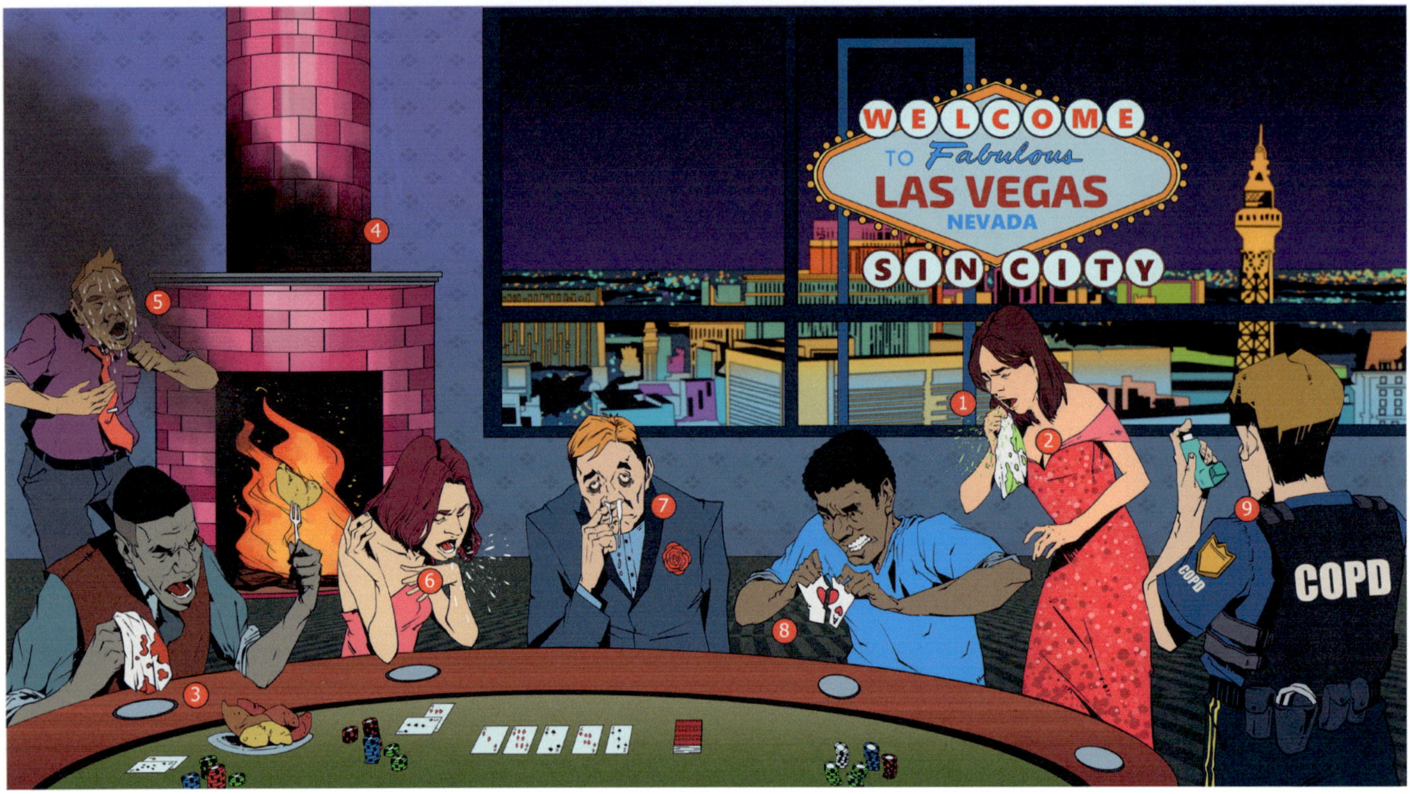

1. Gambler coughing: Cough

2. Green tissue: Sinusitis

3. Tubers and bloody tissue: Tuberculosis

4. Sooted lower portion of the pink rounded chimney: GERD

5. Feverish, sweaty, and coughing employee: Pneumonia

6. Smoke causing gambler to sneeze: URI

7. Runny nose from a flower on tuxedo: Allergic rhinitis

8. Gambler ripping Ace of hearts: ACE inhibitors

9. Colorado police department officer using inhaler: Asthma/COPD

Differential Diagnosis | Section 7 - Shortness of Breath Differential

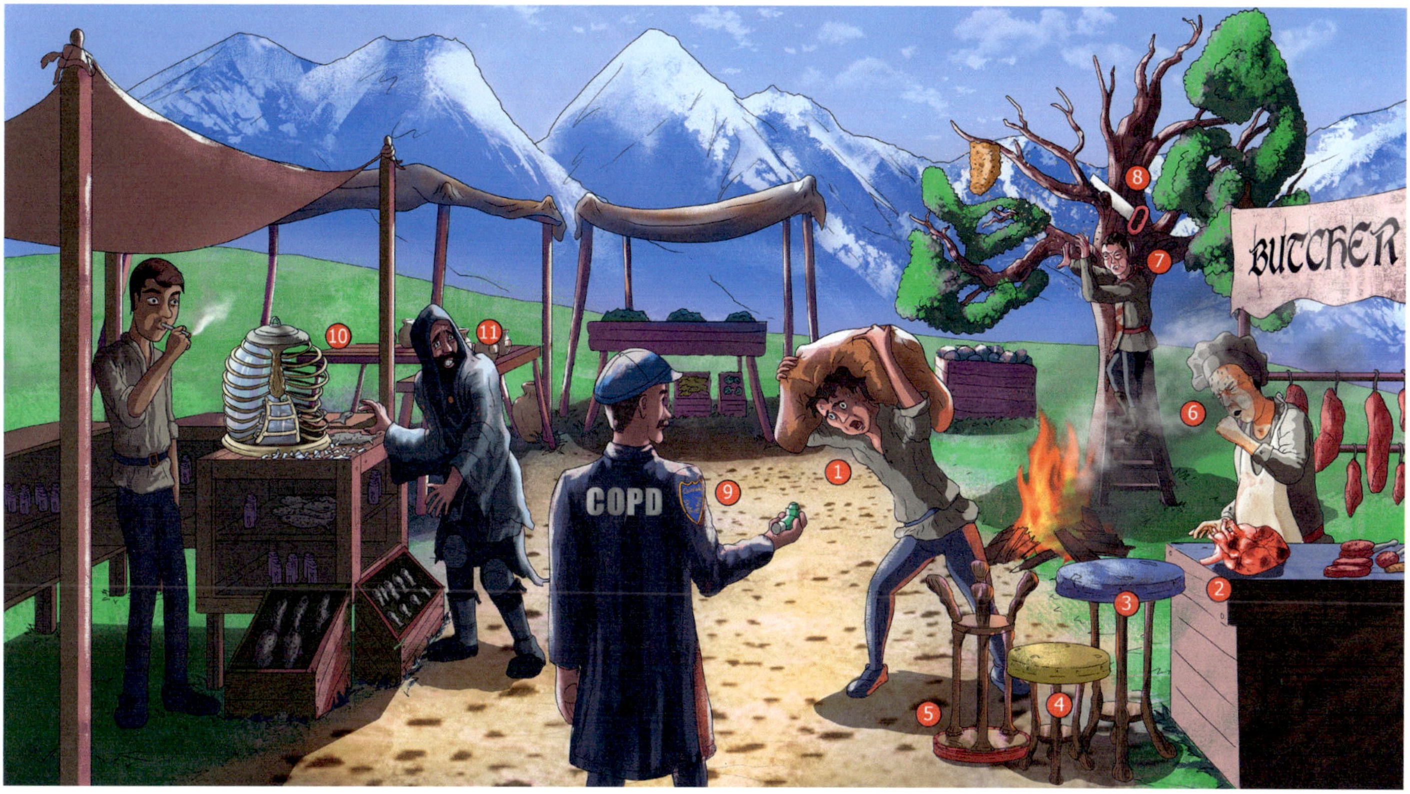

1. Man struggling to breath: Shortness of breath

2. Black unhealthy Bison heart: Acute coronary syndrome

3. Tall STool: ST elevation

4. Short STool: ST depression

5. Upside down stool: Inverted T-wave

6. Butcher coughing and sweating from the hot smoke: Pneumonia

7. Apprentice having an allergic reaction to bees: Anaphylaxis

8. Saw stuck in a branch of a lung-shaped tree: Pulmonary embolism

9. Colorado police department officer using inhaler: COPD/Asthma

10. Air inside a broken thorax-shaped fish tank: Pneumothorax

11. Scared, breathless, anxious thief: Anxiety

Differential Diagnosis | Section 8 - Chest Pain Differential

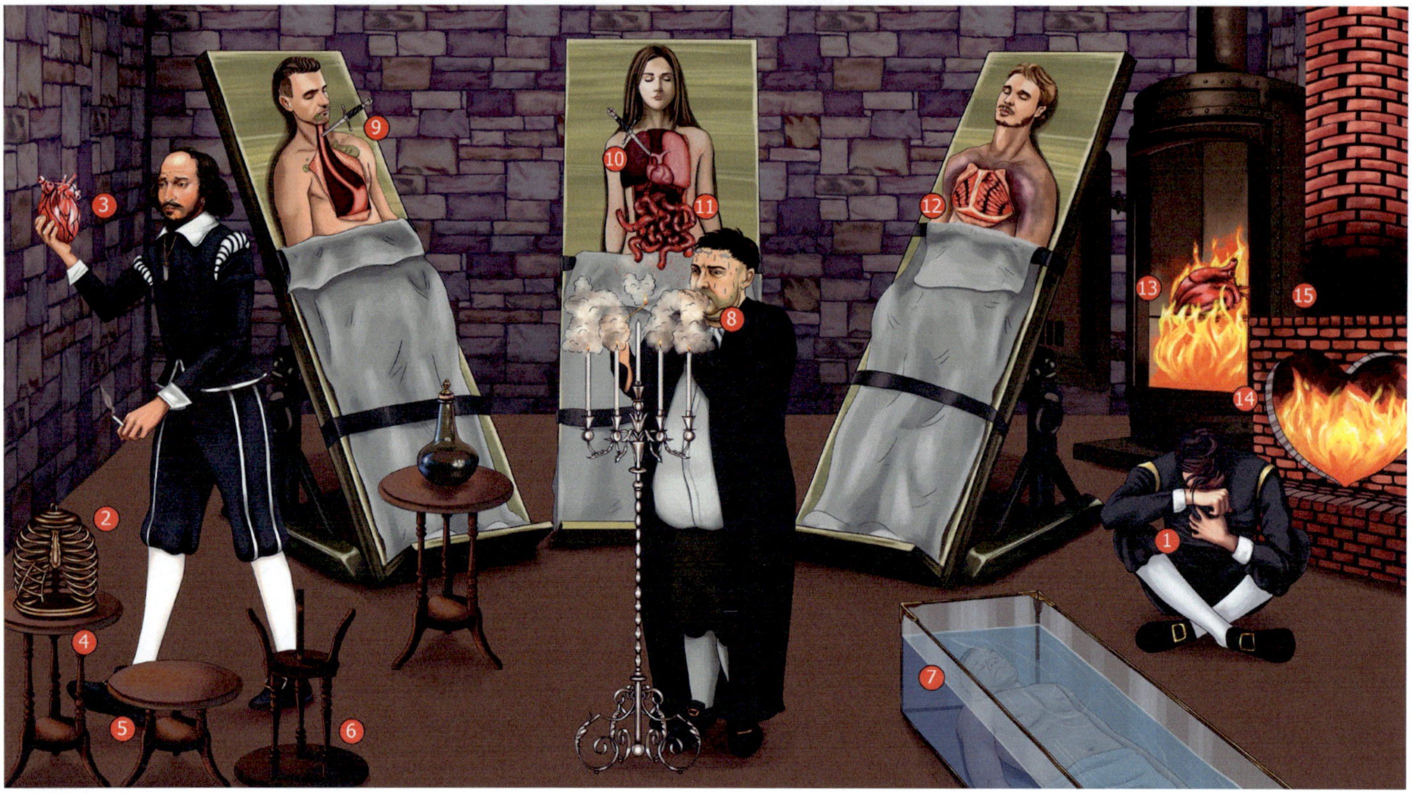

1. Man clutching chest in grief: Chest pain

2. Birdcage shaped like thorax: Pneumothorax

3. Battered-looking heart with black streaks: Acute coronary syndrome

4. Tall STool: ST elevation

5. Short STool: ST depression

6. Inverted stool: Inverted T-wave

7. Cocaine in necklace vial: Cocaine abuse

8. Corpse in a tank of water: Cardiac tamponade

9. Coroner coughing, sweating, and struggling to breathe: Pneumonia

10. Knife lodged in the neck: Esophageal rupture

11. Knife lodged in lung vessels: Pulmonary embolism

12. Chaotic dissection: Aortic dissection

13. Ragged and torn muscles: Musculoskeletal issues

14. Flames around the heart: Pericarditis

15. Flames inside a heart-shaped hearth: Endocarditis

16. Charred bottom of chimney: GERD

Differential Diagnosis | Section 9 - Vomiting Differential

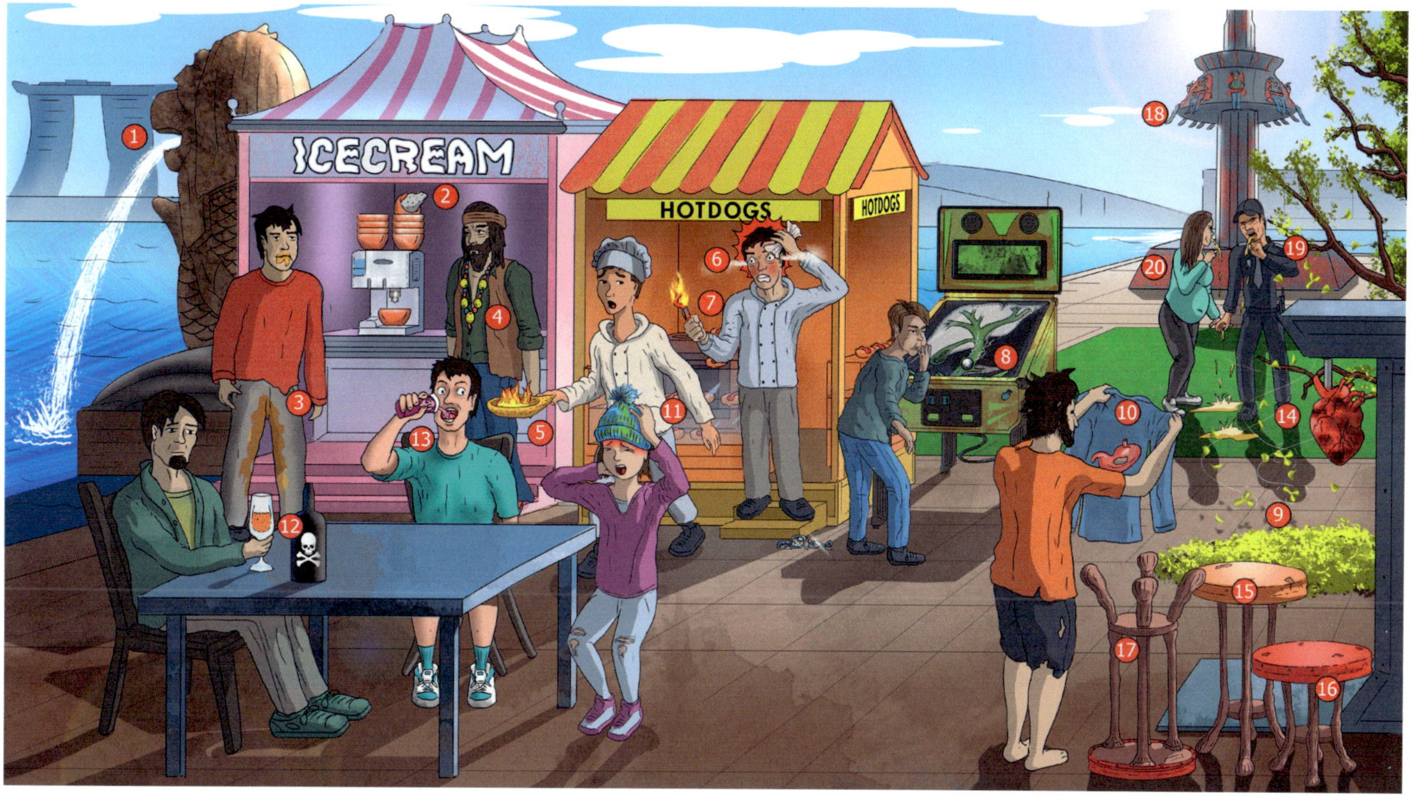

1. Merlion fountain statue spouting water: Vomiting

2. Big stone in the small bowl: Small bowel obstruction

3. Vomit and diarrhea: Acute gastroenteritis

4. Dyed beads with lemon: Diabetic ketoacidosis

5. Flamed pancreas Pan: Pancreatitis

6. Steam coming out of head: Elevated intracranial pressure

7. A pen on fire: Appendicitis

8. Cracked gallbladder pinball machine: Gallbladder and biliary tract diseases

9. Helicopter seeds piling up: Peptic ulcer disease

10. Hole in stomach sweater: Perforated peptic ulcer

11. Tightly fitting green beanie: Meningitis

12. Alcohol and the skull and crossbones bottle: Alcohol and toxins

13. Concentrated electrolyte mix: Abnormal electrolytes

14. Heart-shaped punching bag with black streaks: Acute coronary syndrome

15. Tall STool: ST elevation

16. Short STool: ST depression

17. Inverted stool: Inverted T-wave

18. Vertical drop tower ride: Vertigo

19. Man coughing and vomiting: Post-tussive vomiting

20. Pregnant woman vomiting: Hyperemesis gravidarum

Differential Diagnosis | Section 10 - Upper Abdominal Pain Differential

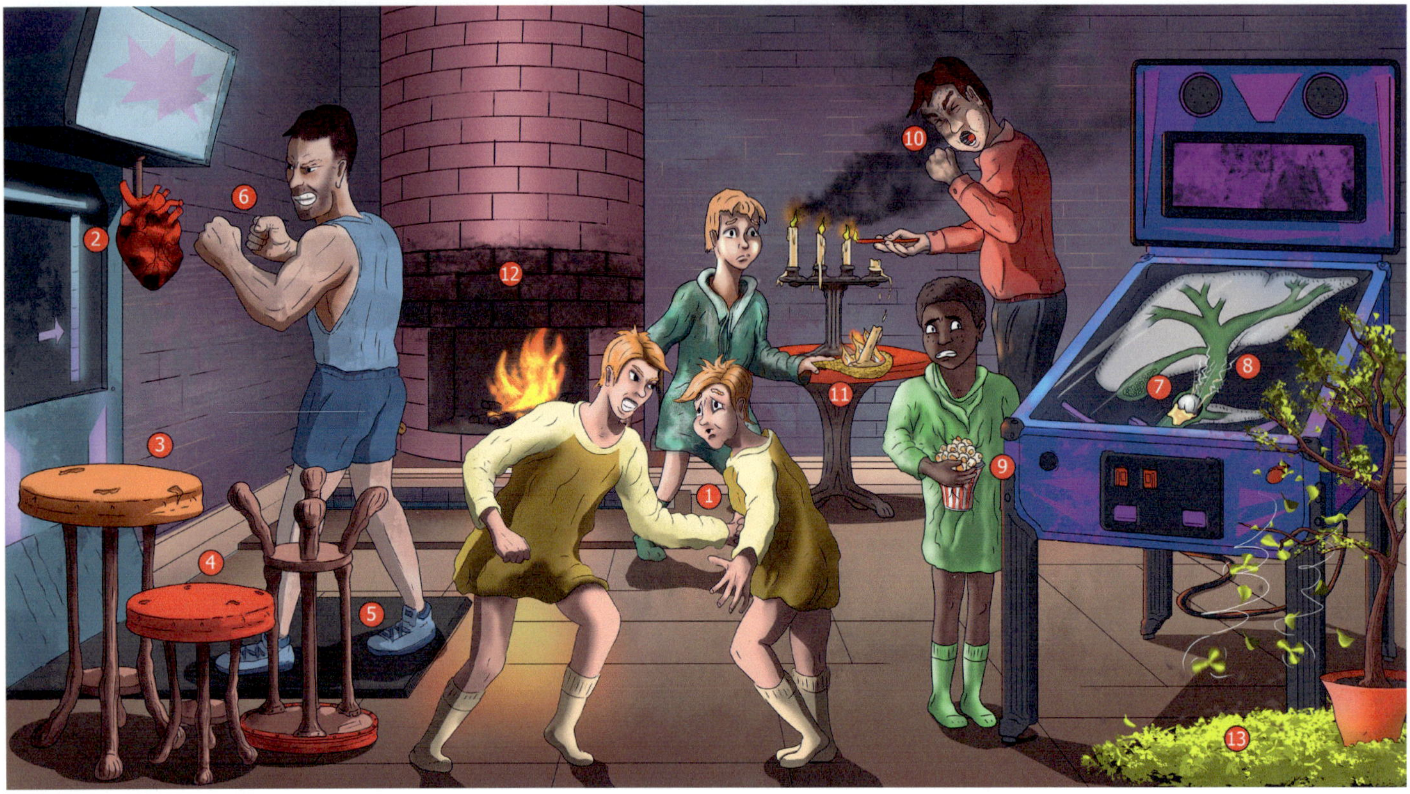

1. Boy getting punched in the upper abdomen: Upper abdominal pain

2. Heart-shaped punching bag with black marks: Acute coronary syndrome

3. Tall STool: STEMI

4. Short STool: Non-STEMI

5. Inverted stool: Inverted T-wave

6. "Huge guy making fists to crush": Fitz-Hugh-Curtis syndrome

7. Lodged ball in biliary tree pinball machine: Biliary colic

8. Cracks and oil on biliary pinball machine: Acute cholangitis

9. Boy pressing his URQ with a yellow cholesterol-shaped popcorn bucket: Cholecystitis

10. Coughing, sweating, and high temperature from candles smoke: Pneumonia

11. Flamed pancreas shaped pan: Pancreatitis

12. Sooted lower portion of pinkish chimney: GERD

13. Pile of helicopter seeds: Peptic ulcer disease

Differential Diagnosis | Section 11 - Diffuse Abdominal & Flank Pain Differential

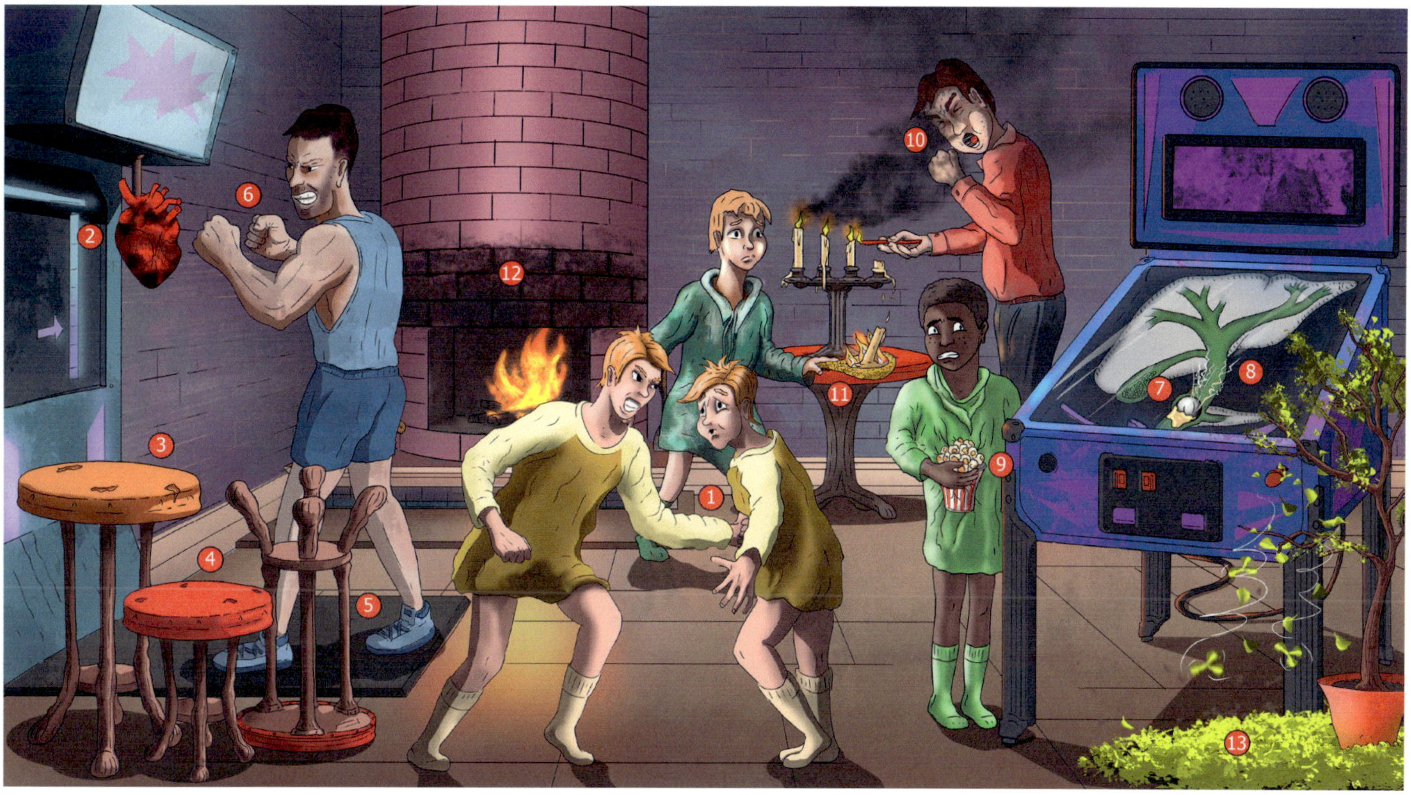

1. Sore red abdomen and flank: Diffuse abdominal and flank pain

2. Exploding triple-A battery: Abdominal aortic aneurysm (AAA)

3. Man wearing dyed beads drinking a lemon shake and syrup: Diabetic ketoacidosis (DKA)

4. Clogged red hose causing the colon tree arch leaves to fall off: Mesenteric ischemia

5. Leaks in the colon-shaped balloon arch: Perforated viscus

6. Small bowls with a large rock inside: Small bowel obstruction (SBO)

7. Man vomiting with diarrhea: Acute gastroenteritis

8. Kidney-shaped stone hitting a passer-by in the flank: Kidney stones

9. Flaming pipes: Pyelonephritis

10. Question mark on abdomen: Non-specific abdominal pain

Differential Diagnosis | Section 12 - Lower Abdominal Pain Differential

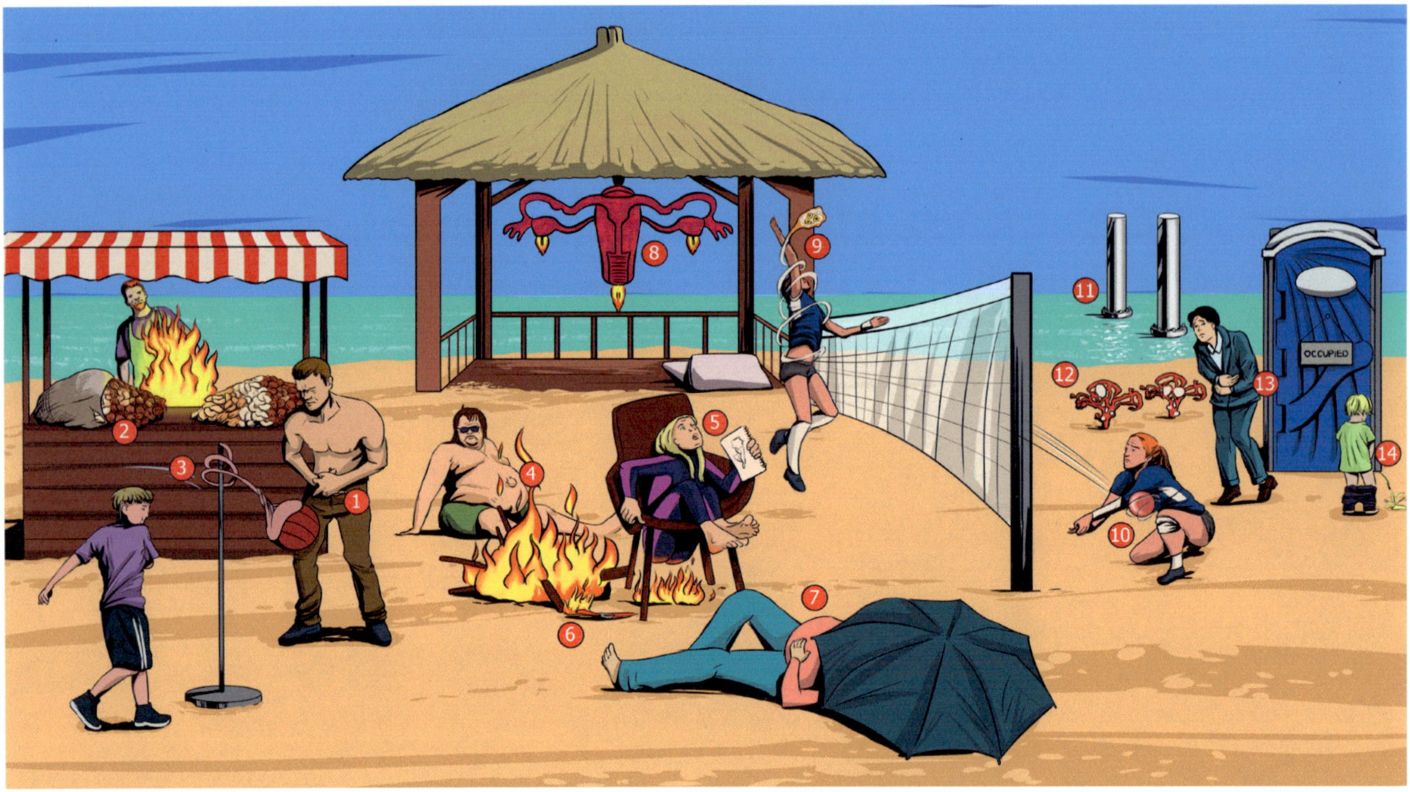

1. Man clutching abdomen in pain below his umbilicus: Lower abdomen pain

2. Roasting bag of nuts: Orchitis/Epididymitis

3. Testis-shaped tetherball rope twisting around the pole: Testicular torsion

4. Obese man with bulges: Hernia

5. Diver's butt bulging out of the seat: Diverticulitis

6. A pen on fire: Appendicitis

7. A pregnant woman half covered by the umbrella: Ectopic pregnancy

8. Female reproductive-shaped chandelier with candles:PID/Tubo-ovarian abscess

9. Ovary-shaped tetherball twisted around the girl: Ovarian torsion

10. Pink, shiny, and semi-translucent volleyball hitting belly: Ovarian cyst

11. Metal poles shimmering on water: Mittelschmerz pain

12. Uterus shaped corals with sand masses: Fibroid

13. A guy holding belly with closed porta-potty: Constipation

14. Boy peeing: UTI

Differential Diagnosis | Section 13 - Back Pain Differential

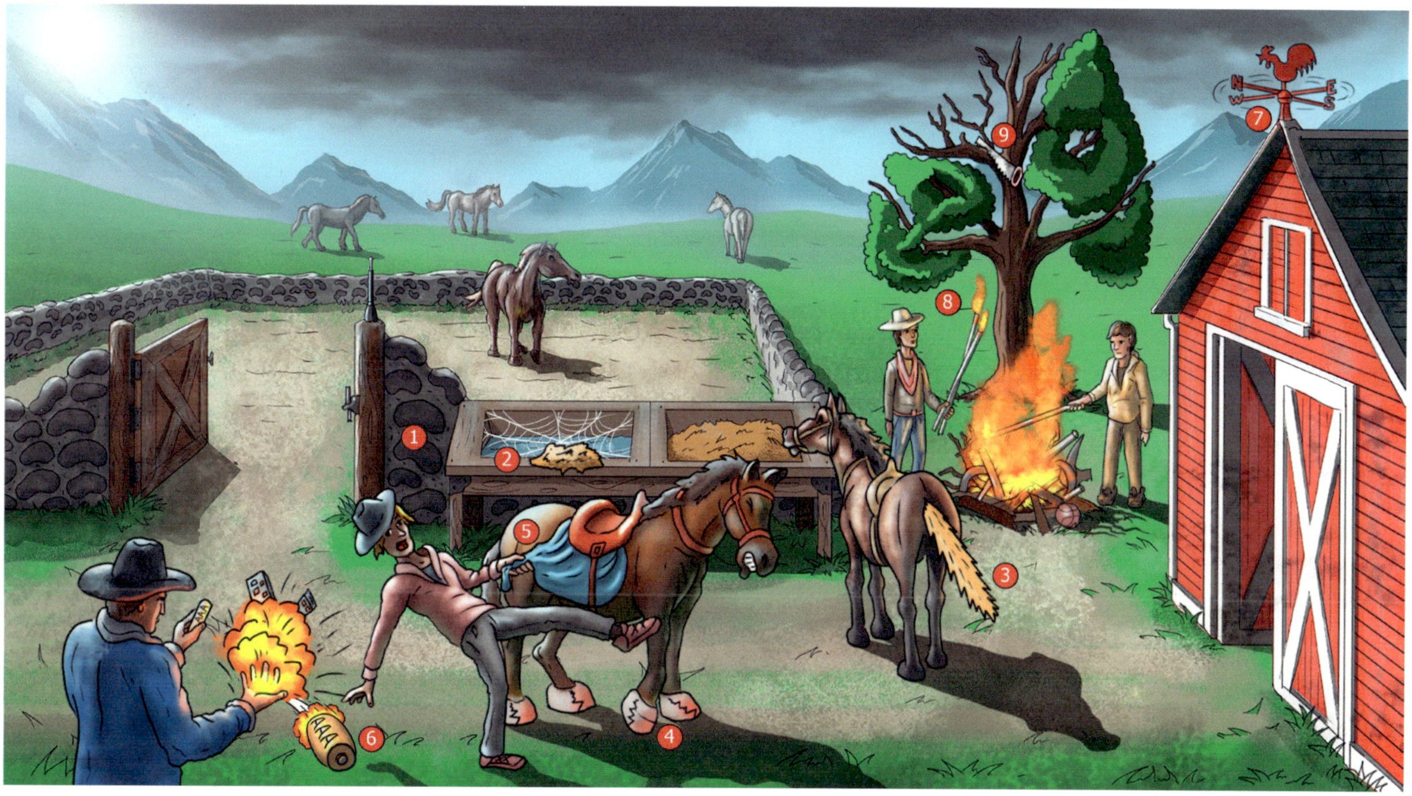

1. Kidney-shaped stones: Kidney stones

2. Food on edge of trough with spider web: Epidural abscess

3. Horse's tail: Cauda equina syndrome

4. Cracked vertebra-shaped hooves: Vertebral compression fractures

5. Cushion being pulled: Intervertebral disk herniation

6. Exploded AAA battery flying away: Abdominal aortic aneurysm

7. Weathercock spinning in storm: Non-specific causes

8. Pipes on fire: Pyelonephritis

9. Lung-shaped tree with a saw lodged in the dead part: Pulmonary embolism

Differential Diagnosis | Section 14 - Leg Pain Differential

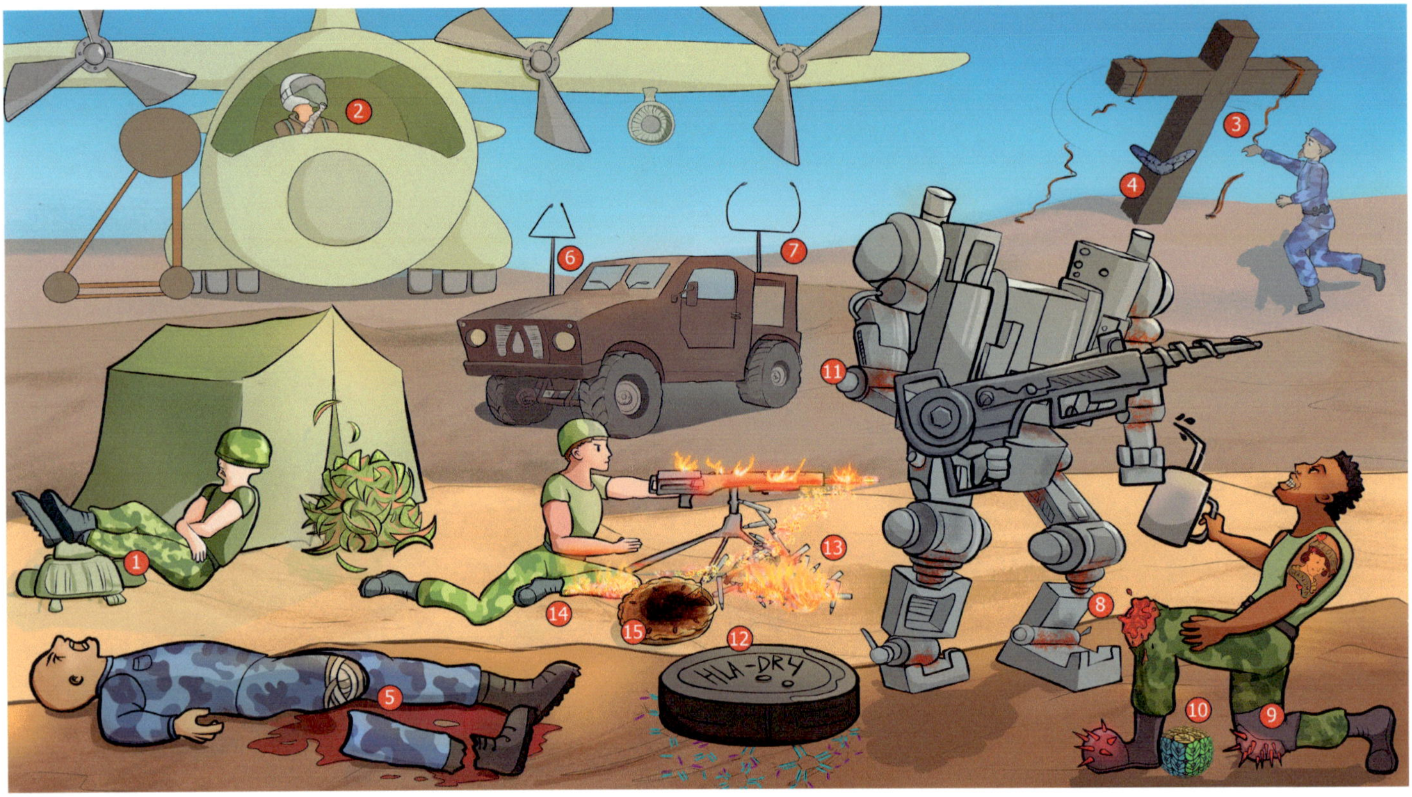

1. Soldier's sore legs: Leg pain

2. Pilot who has been flying for hours: DVT

3. Cut ropes and the cross falling forward: Anterior cruciate ligament tear

4. Boomerang with heavy wear and tear: Meniscus tear

5. Severed knee and ankle: Knee and ankle fractures

6. Antenna bowed inward: Valgus deformity (medial collateral ligament)

7. Antenna curved outward: Varus deformity (lateral collateral ligaments)

8. Soldier shot in the knee: Septic arthritis

9. Spiky knee pads: Gouty arthritis

10. Shield wall Rubik's cube: Granuloma (Sarcoid arthritis)

11. Rusted joints on war machine: Osteoarthritis

12. Roomba robot: Rheumatoid arthritis

13. Pile of flaming bullet shells: Skin abscess

14. Soldier's burning leg: Cellulitis/erysipelas

15. Burned pie: Necrotizing fasciitis

Differential Diagnosis | Section 15 - Ankle & Foot Injuries Differential

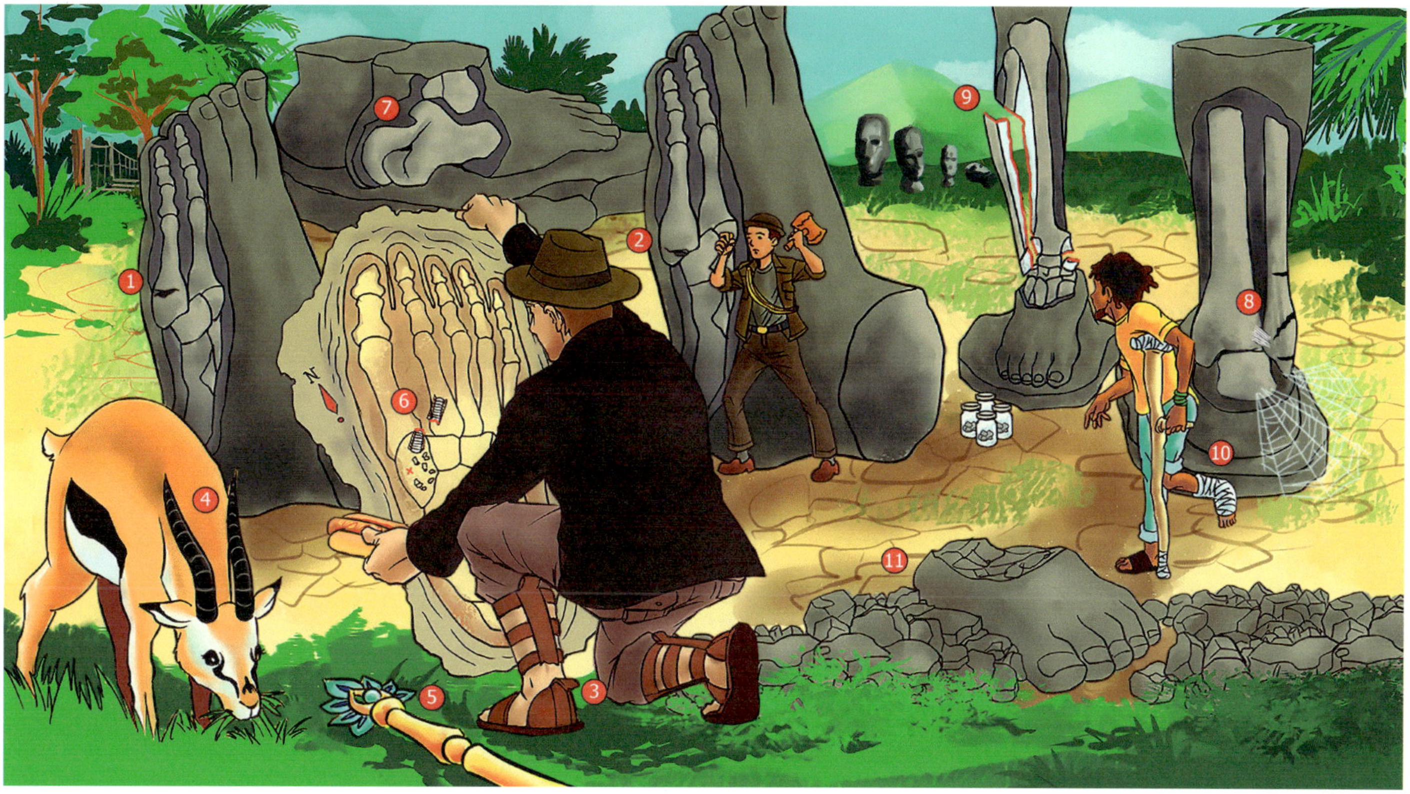

1. Crack being observed by Indiana Jones: Jones fracture

2. Fake Indiana Jones: Pseudo-Jones fracture

3. Torn sandals in area of Achilles tendon: Achilles rupture

4. Thompson gazelle: Positive Thompson test

5. Flower staff: Fluoroquinolones

6. Hot dog or "Franks": Lisfranc injury

7. Cracked heel: Calcaneal fracture

8. Cracked fibula and spider webs below: Weber fractures

9. Cracked statue with Mason jars below: Maisonneuve fracture

10. Guide with wrapped ankle: Ankle sprain

11. Rubble: Other fractures

Differential Diagnosis | Section 16 - Fever Differential

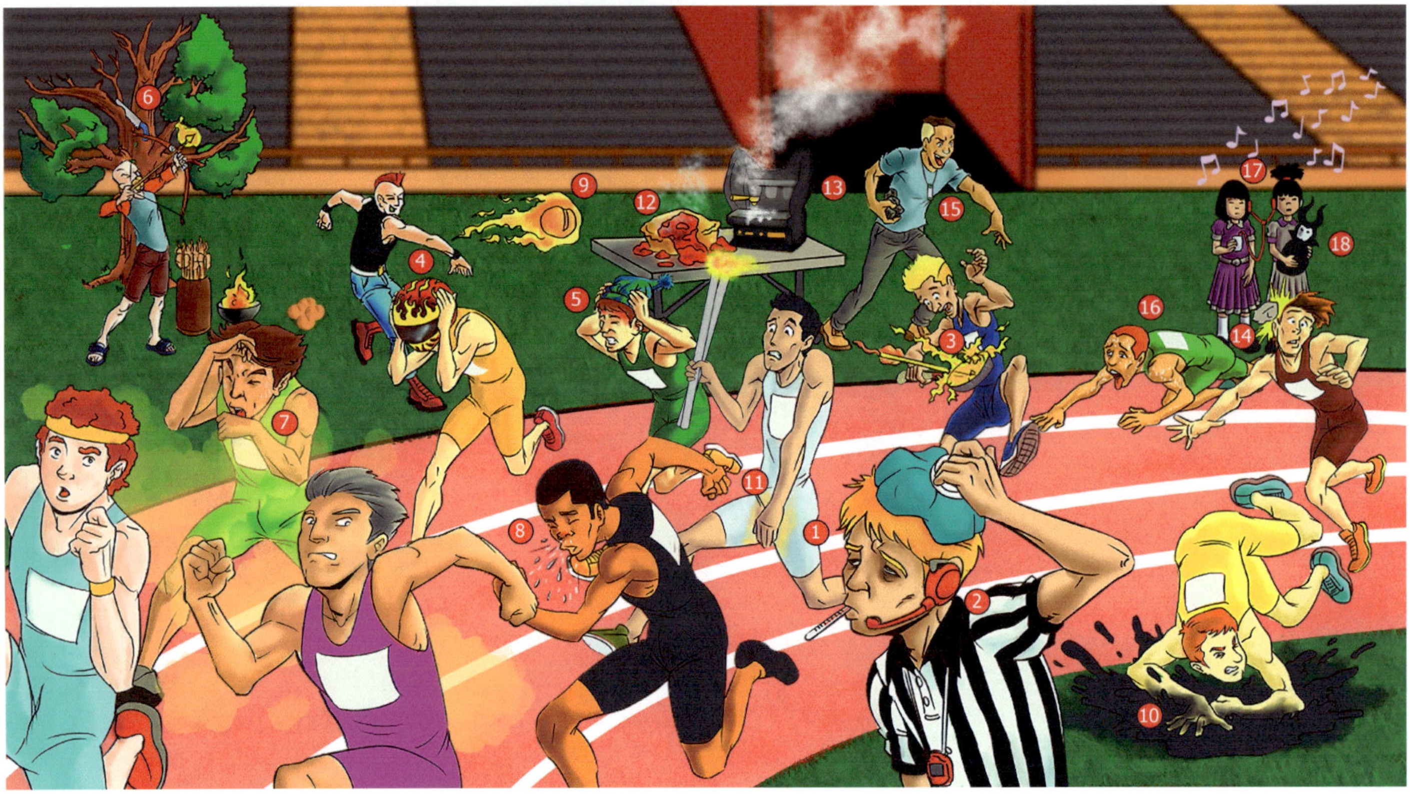

1. Sick referee: Fever

2. Red headset covering the ear: Acute otitis media

3. Flaming arrow with appendix tail hitting pan: Abdominal causes of fever (appendicitis & pancreatitis)

4. Red, flaming helmet: Encephalitis

5. Beanie with greenish spots: Meningitis

6. Lung-shaped tree with a saw wedged proximally to a dead branch: Pulmonary embolism

7. Coughing Runner: Pneumonia

8. Sneezing runner: URI/Viral

9. Flaming prostate-shaped shot put ball: Prostatitis

10. Mud covered skin: Skin infections

11. Urine-soaked runner holding flaming pipes: UTI/ Pyelonephritis

12. Cherry pie: Strep pyogenes

13. Steaming espresso maker shaped like the thyroid gland: Thyroid storm (Hyperthermia)

14. Rock hitting runner in head: CNS lesions (Hyperthermia)

15. Guy with cocaine necklace: Cocaine (Hyperthermia)

16. Overexerted runner: Heat stroke (Hyperthermia)

17. Girls sharing tunes: Serotonin syndrome (Hyperthermia)

18. Maleficent doll: NMS/MH (Hyperthermia)

Differential Diagnosis | Section 17 - Syncope & Pre-Syncope Differential

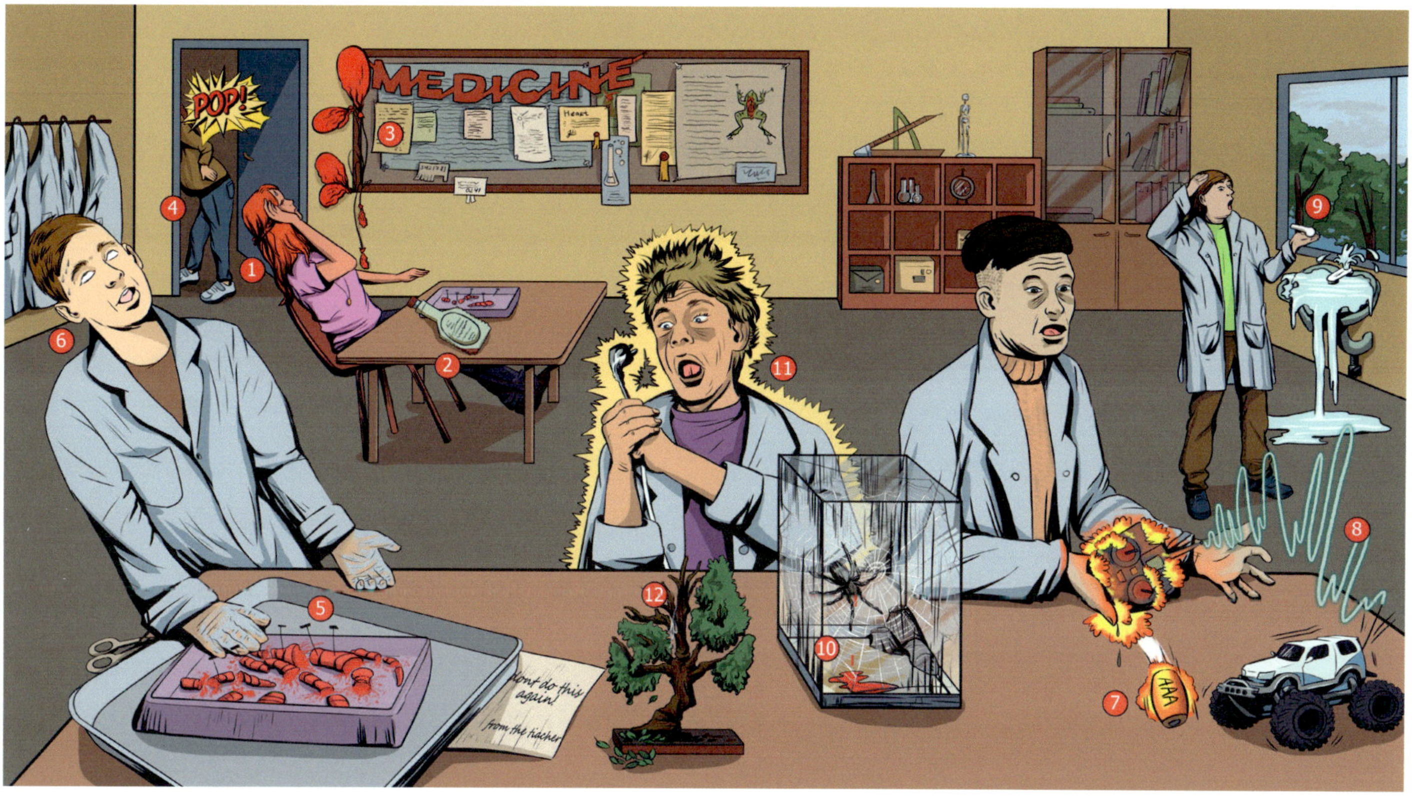

1. Fainting drama queen: Orthostatic hypotension

2. Empty syrup bottle: Hypoglycemia

3. Deflated red balloons: Anemia

4. Popping in the hallway and the pregnant teacher halfway inside: Ectopic rupture

5. Chaotic dissection: Aortic dissection

6. Student sweating with rolled-back eyes: Reflex syncope/vasovagal syncope

7. Exploding triple-A batteries: Abdominal Aortic Aneurysm (AAA) rupture

8. Irregular waves: Cardiac arrhythmias

9. Broken valve of a heart-shaped sink: Cardiac valvular disease

10. Blood puddle under a bleeding arachnid: Subarachnoid hemorrhage

11. Electrocuted shaking student: Seizure

12. Lung shaped tree with a dead branch: Pulmonary embolism

Differential Diagnosis | Section 18 - Weakness Differential

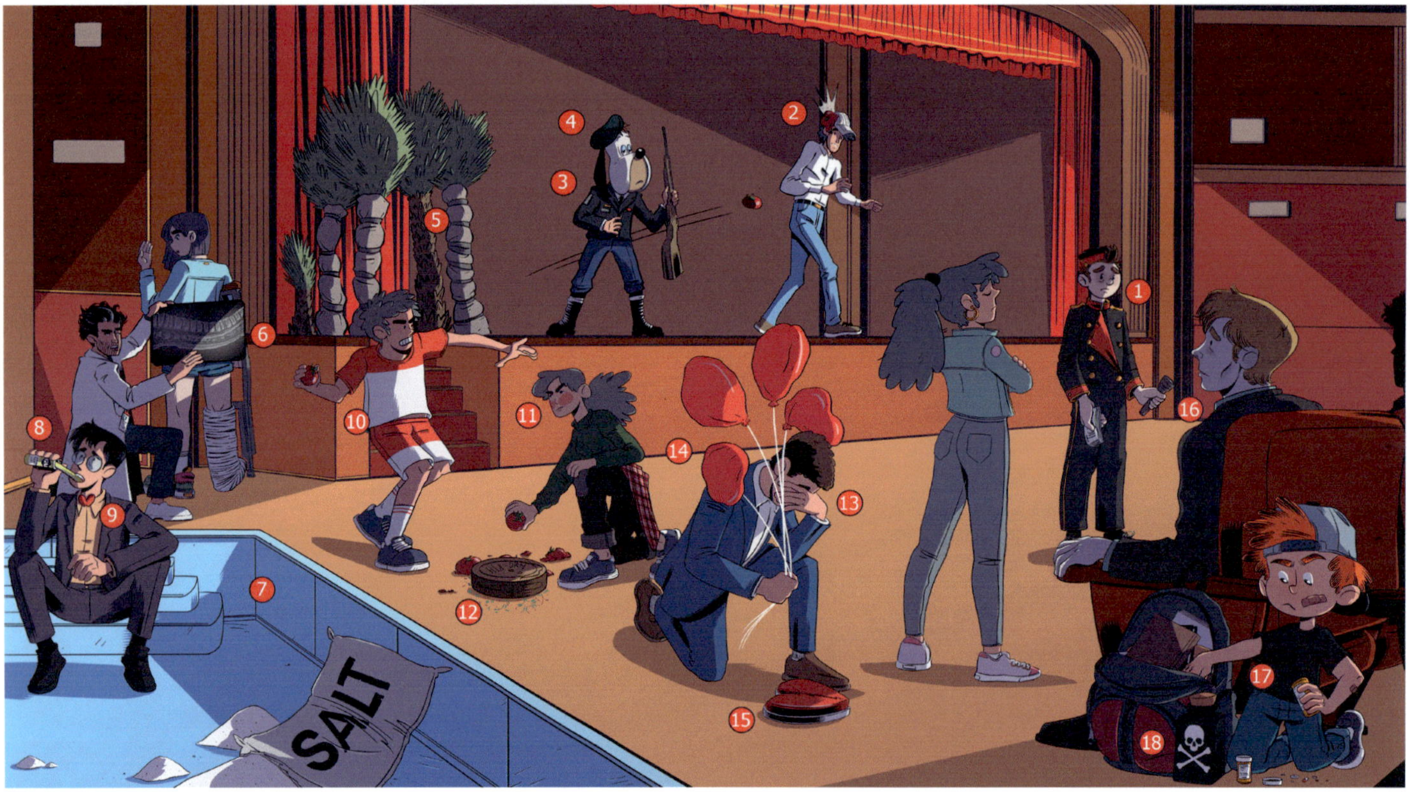

1. Weak usher: Weakness

2. Hit in the head by tomato: Cerebrovascular Accident (Focal weakness)

3. Droopy dog with facial drooping, and ptosis: Myasthenia Gravis (Focal weakness)

4. Green beret: Guillain-Barre syndrome (Focal weakness)

5. Unwrapped palm tree: Multiple sclerosis (Focal weakness)

6. An MRI film held transversely: Transverse myelitis (Focal weakness)

7. Empty pool: Hypovolemia (General weakness)

8. Director chugging concentrated electrolyte mix: Electrolyte imbalance (General weakness)

9. Small bow tie: Hypothyroidism (General weakness)

10. Red proximal areas in the t-shirt and shorts of the upper and lower extremities: Polymyalgia rheumatica (General weakness)

11. Girl with a butterfly-shaped rash on her face: Systemic lupus erythematosus (General weakness)

12. Roomba robot: Rheumatoid arthritis (General weakness)

13. Depressed, rejected man: Depression (General weakness)

14. Deflated red balloon: Anemia (General weakness)

15. Broken heart-shaped chocolate box: Cardiac issues (General weakness)

16. Zombie-like guy: Infections (General weakness)

17. Kid replacing stolen medication with candy: Medication changes (General weakness)

18. Skull and crossbones symbol: Toxins (General weakness)

Differential Diagnosis | Section 19 - Rash Differential

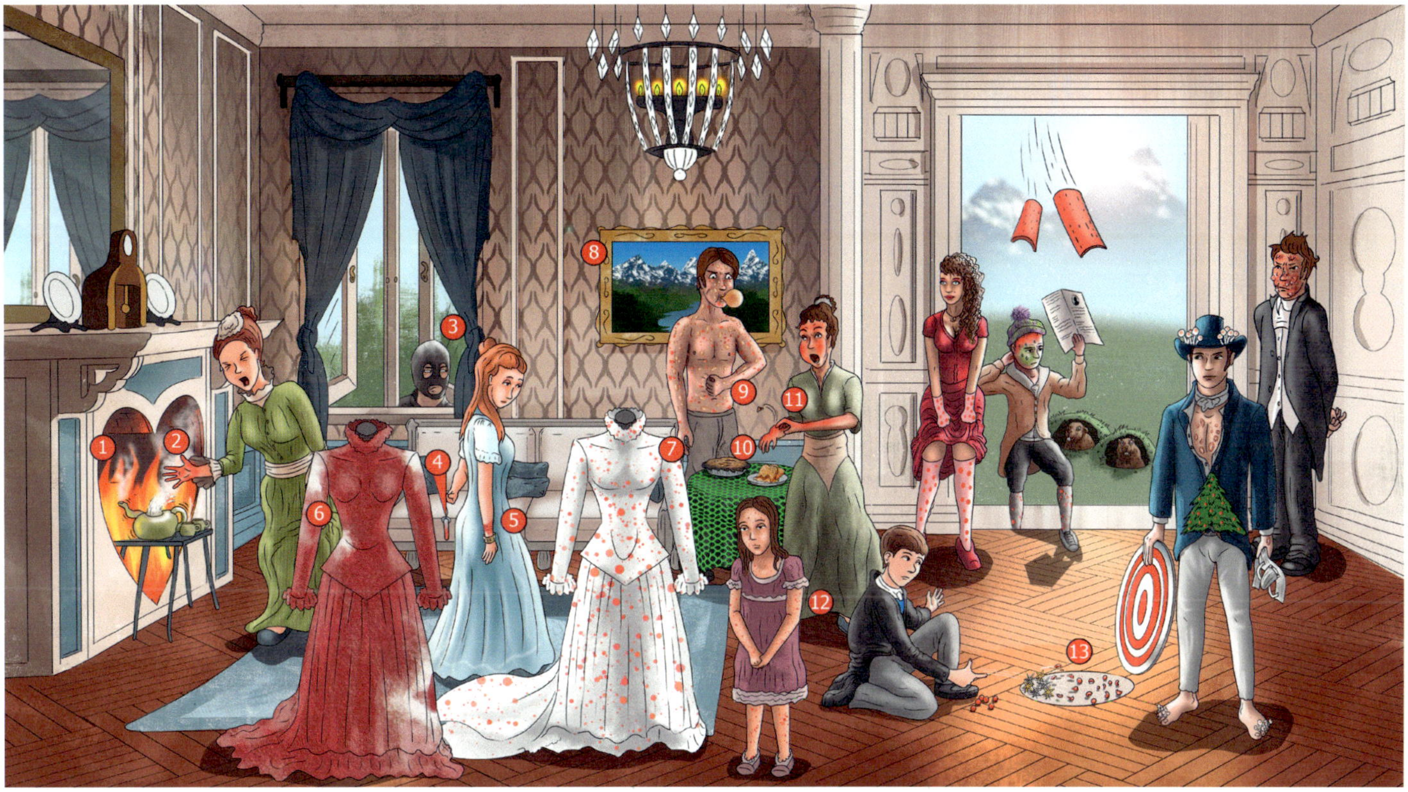

1. Flames inside heart-shaped hearth: Endocarditis

2. Staff member with scalded skin: Staphylococcal scalded skin syndrome

3. Burglar: Lyme Disease (Borrelia burgdorferi)

4. Tampon: Toxic Shock Syndrome

5. Red on the wrist where the bracelet was: Contact dermatitis

6. Red dress with white spots: Erythroderma

7. White dress with red splotches: Dress syndrome

8. Paint of the Rocky Mountains: Rocky Mountain spotted fever

9. Fluorescent fishnet tablecloth and son with blisters: Pemphigus Vulgaris

10. Burnt the pie: Necrotizing fasciitis

11. Swelling after bee sting: Urticaria/Anaphylaxis

12. Young girl with a rash: Viral Exanthem

13. Red marble: Microangiopathic hemolytic anemia (MAHA) (e.g. DIC, TTP)

14. Target: Erythema multiforme

15. Herald with a cluster of lesions on chest: Pityriasis rosea

16. Mushrooms stuck between toes:Tinea infection

17. Mr. Steve Johnson with a red, flushed face: Steven Johnson Syndrome/Toxic epidermal necrolysis

18. Tightly fitting beanie with green splotches: Meningococcemia

19. Red polka dots on girls gloves and stocking: Secondary syphilis

20. Burrowing made by beavers: Scabies infestation

21. Shingles: Shingles (Herpes zoster virus)

Made in the USA
Las Vegas, NV
03 November 2026

57424358R00017